JARM—How To Jog
With Your Arms
To Live Longer

by

Joseph D. Wassersug, M.D.

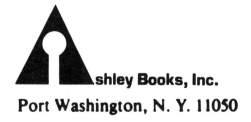

shley Books, Inc.

Port Washington, N. Y. 11050

JARM — How To Jog With Your Arms To Live Longer
(c) Copyright 1984 by Joseph D. Wassersug, M.D.

Library of Congress Number: 81-10919
ISBN: 0-87949-197-3

ASHLEY BOOKS, INC./*Publishers*
Port Washington, New York   11050

Printed in the United States of America
First Edition

9   8   7   6   5   4   3   2   1

Library of Congress Cataloging in Publication Data:

Wassersug, Joseph David, 1912-
   Jarm, how to jog with your arms to live longer.

   Includes bibliographical references and index.
   1. Exercise. 2. Arm. 3. Jogging. 4. Exercise--
Physiological aspects.   I.   Title.
GV508.W37   613.7   81-10919
ISBN   0-87949-197-3   AACR2

Author's Foreword

The author wishes to express his thanks and appreciation to Jordan Abeshouse, M.F.A., Yale Art School, for the fine drawings that illustrate the exercises and activities described in this book. Mr. Abeshouse is Supervisor of Art in Wallingford, Connecticut, and is a renowned portraitist.

In the *appendix* of the book are several drawings adopted by the author from various sources to indicate some of the *anatomical* relationships described in the text. Some, from an old volume of Gray's Anatomy, are included for historical as well as anatomical interest.

To Joshua and Benjamin
and Nathan and Beth

Introduction

You just came in from your daily jogging session. You did your leg-stretching exercises before running and now you're doing your cooling-down exercises. You feel healthy, revitalized, virtuous, perhaps pleasantly tired. But what have you forgotten?

Or you've done your sit-ups, leg kicks and knee bends. Your exercise session is over for the day. What have you forgotten?

Your *arms!* Of course you don't run with your arms or use your arms for knee bends or leg kicks, but that doesn't mean they're less important to your health than your legs. In fact, exercising your arms may significantly improve your general well-being and mental outlook and may also promote longevity.

Arm exercising is not yet as "in" or as popular as jogging. It may not seem as vigorous or energetic as running or other forms of leg exercise. It may not produce weight loss or muscle-firming benefits as quickly. But it *is* crucial to your health and your hopes for a long life.

In this era of holistic health and whole-body consciousness, many people who exercise faithfully (and some physicians) have overlooked the arms. Yet studies show and my own practice confirms the fact that the use of the arms in work or exercise produces many of the same benefits as—without the liabilities of—running.

As a specialist in Internal Medicine, I see an average of thirty patients each day. Of these patients, quite a number jog or exercise routinely. A few patients do arm exercises. And I've seen too many who take no exercise at all. While those patients who exercise or run are generally more fit and happier than those who don't, I was constantly surprised by the overall good condition and age of those who regularly use or exercise their arms.

I began to investigate the subject of arm exercises (what I call *jarming*) and its relation to health and longevity. I have been very pleased with my findings and now prescribe arm exercises for most of my patients. I do them too, every day. Whether our life spans will be lengthened or not remains to be seen, but right now I'm enjoying life and I've never felt better.

Isn't a healthier, happier, longer life worth a few minutes of your time each day? You'll find my simple exercises pleasant and invigorating. Come on and heed the rallying cry of the truly physically fit—To arms! To jarms!

JARM—How To Jog With Your Arms To Live Longer

CHAPTER I

What Arm Jogging Can Do For You

People who work with or exercise their arms live longer and healthier lives than sedentary individuals or those who primarily use their legs in their day's work or play. This is true throughout the world, in all cultures and societies, in all classes and economic groups.

Take window washers, for example. They almost never die, nor do they fade away. Two of our patients were partners in a window-washing business. One lived into his mid-nineties, despite a bout of severe pneumonia a few years earlier. The other died in his late eighties, having survived the insertion of two consecutive cardiac pacemakers. These men had been professional window-washers, cleaning office building windows on ladders and scaffolding. All their lives they had used their arms vigorously, with speed and skill, to earn their livelihood.

They were fine, vigorous, alert men until their deaths.

Or consider King Christian of Denmark who played tennis until his late eighties, conductor Arturo Toscanini who died at ninety, and Leopold Stokowski who lived until his ninety-fifth birthday. What's the connection between these famous men and our window-washing patients? They all worked or played vigorously with their arms and hands.

Although doctors have recently begun to recognize the fact that symphony conductors live longer than most individuals, they have failed to come up with a simple answer to account for this remarkable phenomenon. For example, at the University of California's San Diego School of Medicine, Dr. Donald H. Atlas found that maestros live an average of 73.4 years as compared to 68.5 years for the average American male. Among other notable examples he cites Bruno Walter who died at eighty-five and Walter Damrosch who lived to the age of eighty-eight.

Dr. Atlas, however, is at a loss for a simple explanation for the remarkable longevity of symphony conductors. "These maestros," he reports, "remained musically productive and generally active in all phases of life virtually to the actual moment of death." He postulates that while stress may be injurious to ordinary coronary-prone celebrities, the "gratifying stress" that symphony conductors must feel may have the opposite effect. He believes that the superior intelligence, musical talent or genius, driving motivation, and, most importantly, the sense of fulfillment received from world recognition are common to these conductors and may explain their longevity.

But the great Austrian conductor Karl Bohm, who recently, at the age of eighty-four, conducted the three-hour Beethoven classic *"Fidelio"* at the Metropolitan

Opera, was more to the point. When queried about the vigors of conducting, Bohm said, "Moving your arms around for several hours — I would like to see how long a young man, who is not used to swinging a baton, can stand this!"

Please note and remember every word! Karl Bohm conducted his first opera in 1917, and since then has conducted over 160 operas throughout the world. He says his stamina is not a result of any special mystique from some subtle genius or hypothetical resistance to stress. His stamina derives from a source that is available to each and every one of us — *swinging a baton!* His strength and stamina come from the constant practice of using his arms. But you don't have to be a famous conductor to use your arms. With arm jogging you can develop the longevity and stamina of the most famous opera conductors in the world. You don't even need an education in music.

Arthur Fiedler, conductor of the Boston Pops Orchestra, was a prime example of the therapeutic value of arm jogging. At the age of eighty-four he underwent major brain surgery. A few months later he was able to conduct the Boston Pops Orchestra with almost his usual skill and agility. Many doctors are convinced the Fiedler's arm exercise, carried on through his entire life, was the most important factor in his speedy recovery from brain surgery at such an advanced age.

In subsequent chapters we shall discuss many easy arm exercises which anyone can do. We shall comment on the current destructive fad of (leg) jogging and talk about the many advantages arm jogging has over leg jogging. We shall discuss the greater physiologic and spiritual benefits of arm exercises over leg exercises.

For the present it is enough to say that there is an

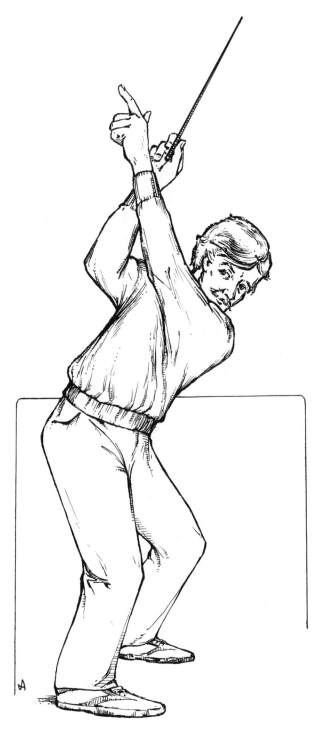

almost untold wealth of benefits to be gained from a program of arm exercises. Just think a moment. Did you ever wonder why so many of the ancient Oriental gods are depicted as sitting quietly on their crossed legs while their arms (often two or three pairs of them) move up and down from the shoulder girdle? Was there something about arm exercises that the Oriental gods learned long ago which mankind has since forgotten? Is there a *physical* as well as spiritual message here?

Before we get into the specifics of arm exercises, let us consider in the next chapter leg jogging, its advantages and disadvantages. We shall see why the fad of leg jogging is running itself out and we will see, in later chapters, why arm jogging is about to replace it.

CHAPTER II

WHAT RUNNING AND JOGGING DO TO YOU

Running and jogging are good for your heart and circulation if, of course, your heart and circulation can take the strain. Running and jogging also strengthen your leg muscles *if* your legs have no inherent structural or physiologic weakness and *if* you are lucky or rich enough to have a good pair of running shoes. Running may also be spiritually rewarding because it makes you feel "good" and even "ecstatic," but devotees of quiet Zen meditation, periodic fasting, or vegetarianism report equal spiritual rewards.

There is no question that the jogging craze has captured the minds and hearts of many people. According to Steven I. Subotnick, D.P.M., a professor of podiatry at the California College of Podiatric Medicine in San Francisco, between 25 and 30 million Americans jog every day putting a lot of stress on their feet which he calls "the weakest link in the runner's anatomy."

A recent issue of *Emergency Medicine* calls attention to the fact that jogging has reached epidemic proportions and tells doctors they must be aware of the effect that running has on the entire body so they can safely prescribe exercise and treat any strains and disorders that occur.

Most people are unaware of the huge physical strain that results from running. Yet, according to Dr. Wayne B. Leadbetter, a member of the American College of Sports Medicine, "The cumulative impact of the feet hitting the ground in running is staggering. Consider that in walking the force load on the ankle joint is five times body weight and at the hip and knee it's roughly three times. In running, the marked increase in this force will unmask any structural weaknesses the runner may have. The effect of impact on an individual runner will vary directly with body weight, distance run, shock absorption of his shoes, and type of running surface."[1]

Assuming a normal *circulation* to the legs (no significant arteriosclerosis, phlebitis or clots) and a normal *nerve* supply (no polio, MS, or other neurologic disorder), a good understanding of the bones and muscles of the leg is essential to the would-be jogger.

The thigh bone is the *femur.* It is the longest, biggest bone in the body in the body and it hooks into the pelvis (acetabulum) in a smooth, well-lubricated ball-and-socket joint. The strength of the hip is illustrated by the athlete who kicks a football a hundred yards down the field. The versatility of the hip joint is demonstrated by the dancer who does a split in one second and then in another kicks higher than her head.

The knee joint is a *hinge,* like the hinge on your door, not a ball and socket. It moves efficiently in only one plane, back and forth, not around and around. Any instability of the knee can strain the ligaments and tendons and even damage the cartilage that lines this joint. Instability of this joint can be the result of such simple things as obesity or flat feet. For example, sneakers that don't support the arch of the foot tend to cause a flattening of the arch with resulting pronation and turning outward of the toes. As the toes turn out the inner aspect of the knees is strained. In time there may be thickening of the knee joint and even arthritis. Any runner who forgets that the knee is a hinge is in for trouble.

In the lower leg there are two bones, the *tibia* and the *fibula*. The tibia is the bigger and stronger of the two and it supports the inner calf muscles. The fibula is a fragile bone. It plays no role in forming the knee joint but it helps give support to the ankle. At the ankle it is easily chipped or fractured by sudden twists and turns.

The ankle joint consists of the tibia, the fibula and a foot bone called the *talus*. From the jogger's standpoint the more important foot bones are the *metatarsals* and the *calcaneus* or heel bone. Jogging can fracture a metatarsal bone. Spurs on the heel can hurt like a piece of imbedded glass. Toes can be injured, especially if jogging shoes are too tight.

Three sets or pairs of muscles are important to the jogger. Three large muscles are toward the front of the body and three are to the rear. Uppermost and in front are the abdominal muscles that hold firm the abdominal wall. Toward the back, securing the lower spine, are the psoas muscles which provide strength to the back in flexion and extension motions. A runner can't run without holding his abdominal muscles and back firm and straight and it is these muscles that are the primary source of energy and stability in the trunk area.

The thigh is kept steady and active by the *quadriceps*

muscles in front and the *hamstring* muscles in back. They extend along the whole length of the femur from the hip to the knee. Pulls or tears of the hamstring muscles are not uncommon with strenuous exercise or exertion. Quadriceps setting exercises to strengthen the legs can be carried out even if the patient is lying down or immobilized. The quadriceps muscles and the hamstrings work in tandem to keep the hips and knees aligned and smoothly functioning.

In the lower leg are the *pretibial* muscles in front and the *calf* muscles in the rear. The pretibial muscles are more related to functioning of the ankle; the calf muscles attach to the knee above and, by the Achilles tendon, to the heel below. Sore calf muscles are common in beginning joggers.

The main blood supply to the legs comes off the lower aorta where it divides into a right and left *iliac* artery which then descends into each leg as the *femoral* artery. There are also comparable iliac and femoral *veins* to pick up and transport the returning blood.

Any obstruction or blocking of these arteries can cause severe leg pain. In advanced cases, especially in older persons, a blocked artery that cannot be bypassed by a graft may lead to gangrene of a foot or leg and possible amputation. While the leg arteries are large and powerful, they are more liable to arteriosclerosis and blockage than arm arteries. One of the great advantages that arm jogging has over running is the fact that it is very difficult to block an arm artery. Not impossible, but very difficult.

"How does your body run?" asks Dr. William L. Haskell, Assistant Professor of Medicine at Stanford University School of Medicine. Dr. Haskell answers his question by stating first that there are two kinds of exercise: 1) aerobic and 2) anaerobic. The former stimulates the heart, enhances endurance and thus increases the heart's ability to withstand strain. Anaerobic exercise is, like weight lifting, conducive to building strength and muscle mass but actually may have a deleterious effect on the heart, especially if the individual already has high blood pressure or other heart problems. How the body runs deals with *aerobic* exercises.

Everyone agrees that running stimulates the whole body — the heart, the lungs, the entire circulation. But it must also be noted that a brief run that fails to increase the pulse rate or fails to bring on sweating and open the body's pores may be inadequate. To get any real benefit from running, you have to put real effort into it.

Your heart can speed up slightly even *before* the running starts. Your heart seems to know what your brain is thinking and the heart may get started "running" even before you do. Once running starts, breathing speeds up. The normal rate of breathing of 10 to 12 liters per minute can increase to about 120 liters per minute during strenuous exercise.

During running, the muscles need both extra blood and extra oxygen. As running progresses and as the breathing and heart rate speed up, the blood vessels respond to the increased metabolism and the arteries and veins in the muscles dilate. More blood goes in and out of the muscles and more blood circulates through the heart and lungs. Even blood flow to the skin increases (by as much as 15 percent) and sweating begins in the attempt to dissipate the increased heat. Both the rate and the force of the heart increase too and there is an accompanying increase in cardiac output.

One of the alleged benefits of running is that it enhances cardiac output and thus, improves the "efficien-

21

cy" of the heart and coronary vessels. Most of the evidence indicates that supervised or regulated running is beneficial to the heart if the heart can stand the strain.

According to Dr. William L. Haskell: "To produce a change in cardiovascular function thought to be associated with some kind of health improvement or reduction in risk of heart disease, a patient must exercise at around 60 to 75 percent of his exercise capacity. Less than that just does not put enough stress on the cardiovascular system to produce much of a training effect. More than that will probably bring fatigue before the exercise does much good and will also expose the patient to greater risks from both the cardiovascular and the orthopedic standpoints."[1]

As Dr. Haskell explains, "It's not the increase in the heart rate itself that produces the training effect, however, but the actual metabolic process needed to increase the heart rate and keep it at that level." The three significant factors in an exercise program are thus: 1) intensity, 2) frequency and 3) duration. In other words, when you start a running program you must warm up or start slowly, train yourself to do a little more each time, and keep the exercise program going and not give up too easily.

Although we made an exhaustive search of the medical records, we could not find any autopsy reports on the hearts of elderly symphony conductors. On the other hand, there are many records available on runners and joggers, even on the famous long-distance runner, Clarence DeMar. Although he had a fairly severe heart condition, he was a many-times winner of the Boston Marathon.

Running, it is now known, thickens the heart wall muscle. This is both an advantage and a disadvantage.

The disadvantage is that the thick muscle wall needs an enhanced coronary blood supply to feed the larger muscle mass. The advantage is that the enlarged runner's heart also performs better. Sometimes it is hard to tell whether the enlargement is normal or abnormal.

Fortunately, tests of heart mass and function can be made nowadays on living runners. Muscle mass can be approximated on regular heart x-rays, yet better evaluated with echo studies and through intravenous injections of radionuclides such as thallium. Function can be further analyzed through measurements taken during stress testing. Electrocardiograms reveal heart rhythms and certain other heart functions. Such tests show that runners not only have slow, large hearts but that there can be significant irregularities in cardiac rhythm. Rhythms that would be considered abnormal in non-runners are sometimes considered normal when they occur in runners. Doctors, even expert cardiologists, have occasionally made mistakes in judging as normal what later proved to be abnormal or even fatal.

Runners are also subject to other potential health problems that are far less likely to occur in arm joggers. The first is water loss and dehydration, a medical problem that runners share with other strenuous laborers or exercisers. According to Dr. Roy H. Maffly, a professor of medicine at Stanford University School of Medicine at Palo Alto, California, "Since sweat consists primarily of water and NaCl, heavy sweating can lead to severe compromise of the function of the entire body." The resulting "massive water and electrolyte shifts. . .can not only impair an athlete's performance but may actually endanger his life."[1] Part of good sport training should include teaching the athlete how to minimize the dangers resulting from water and salt loss. This is especially true of long-distance or marathon runners.

Leg and foot injuries are the most common of the runner's woes. In running, the normal foot contacts the ground on the outside of the heel and then quickly rolls inward or outward depending on the surface. Since the running foot is relatively unstable as the heel contacts the ground, it absorbs the initial stress of contact. But then the heel becomes more stable and it is completely rigid just before toe-off. The mechanical stresses of running are quite complicated. If the foot is abnormal or unstable, strains and injuries result. Proper training can prevent some of these pitfalls.

Sometimes the problem is with the terrian, not with the runner. Both the daydreamer and the inspired or euphoric individual fail to see the pothole before stepping into it. Severe sprains or even fractures of the foot or ankle can result. Strangely, the novice is usually more careful and observant than the experienced runner and is less likely to be injured in this fashion.

The list of possible foot and ankle injuries is seemingly endless. Sprains, muscle tears, joint effusions, heel spurs, nerve injuries, bruises, fallen arches, pulled ligaments — all these and other problems can arise. With care and training, of course, the anticipated benefits of jogging can outweigh the harmful aspects. But with running and jogging the hazards are all there, including such possible dangers as being struck by an automobile or being mugged. These two misfortunes can never happen to the arm jogger.

Finally, there is no *scientific* evidence that jogging or running increases longevity. It has been claimed that such exercise is beneficial to cardiac patients. The evidence is inconclusive however. An equally good or better case has been made for owning a pet such as a dog.

Cardiac patients who own dogs do better, recover more easily, live longer, than those who don't have pets.

---

[1]Roy H. Maffly, "Running Out of Water," *Emergency Medicine*, June 15, 1979, p.57.

CHAPTER III

THE ARMS:
ANATOMY AND PHYSIOLOGY

All mammalian quadripeds and bipeds have legs that are remarkably similar in shape and function, but the human animal has arms and hands that are marvels of anatomic ingenuity. Indeed, many anatomists have postulated that the remarkable development of the brain was a direct consequence of the early simian evolutionary development of a prehensile thumb and the subsequent use of tools. For complexity of form and function, the arm (upper extremity) easily surpasses that of the leg (lower extremity).

Consider for a moment the ingenuity and versatility of the arms and hands. On a macro basis, there is the flying grace and beauty of the trapeze artist, the precision of the professional basketfall player. In art, for example, there is, on one hand, Michelangelo's Sistine Chapel — broadly conceived and broadly executed — and in contrast, the Fabergé Easter eggs, decorated in exquisite miniature figures for Czarist royalty.

Coordination of eye, brain and hand can be illustrated by David's slingshot slaying of Goliath, the rifle marksmanship of a Sergeant York, or the piano virtuosity of Rachmaninoff. The symphony conductor, the violinist, the portrait painter, the key punch operator, the person at the telephone switchboard all demonstrate the remarkable and exquisite diversity of the coordinated function of the arms and hands. Right around you are an almost endless number of similar examples — in the home: sewing, cake decorating; in the factory: assembling barely visible transistors or soldering fine wires; at play: cards, crocheting. On the other hand human legs are good for nothing much other than standing, running, walking, kicking or dancing.

Since the shoulder is a shallow ball-and-socket joint, its range of motion is so broad as to allow 360° in a vertical plane and about 90° in a horizontal plane, plus a fair degree of internal and external rotation. The top of the *humerus* (arm bone), is the ball of the ball-and-socket joint and the *glenoid* cavity of the shoulder blade *(scapula)* is the socket. While the outside of the collarbone *(clavicle)* hooks up to the scapula and provides support and protection to the shoulder, the collarbone is not part of the joint itself.

Dislocations and fractures of the shoulder are not rare occurences since the joint is shallow and, consequently, rather easily disturbed by strains and other traumas. Dislocation results when the joint is forced through an arc exceeding its normal range of motion. Although such dislocations are ordinarily easily "reduced" or repaired, chronic dislocations may need the help of a skilled orthopedic surgeon for operative strengthening of the joint. About the only ways to fracture a shoulder are through a fall or a severe blow to the shoulder itself. We have found no records indicating that orchestra conductors or concert violinists suffer any shoulder disabilities at all from wielding a baton or a bow.

Ligaments and tendons hold the shallow shoulder joint in place. The ligaments are variously called *coracoclavicular* and *coracohumeral* and the main tendons are those that belong to the *biceps* (on the front of the upper arm) and *triceps* (on the back of the upper arm) muscles. Just outside the bones of the joint is a small sac called the *subdeltoid bursa,* cushioned between the muscle layers of the shoulders. It is a common site of inflammation (bursitis) and often a cause of shoulder pain. It's not too hard to "pull" a shoulder tendon, especially the biceps: trying to open a stuck double-hung window by thrusting vigorously from below can often provoke this shoulder injury.

Most important to the arm jogger is the knowledge that the shoulder joint has an excellent nerve and blood supply. The arteries and veins are large and serviceable, lying as they do so close to the heart itself. The main blood vessels are the *brachial* artery and vein, but their branches, such as the *thoraco-acromial,* the *transvere scapular,* and the *scapular circumflex,* form a rich vascular network around the shoulder joint and practically guarantee the joint good nutrition and good oxygenation.

Similarly, the nerves to the shoulder and to the rest of the arm and hand are fused together into a thick bundle that resembles a heavy coaxial cable and the nerves run from the spine and thorax across the armpits to the arm right under the shoulder joint itself. This large cable composed of many individual nerve fibers is the *brachial plexus* and it includes in its bundle such important nerve branches as the *median,* the *radial,* and the *ulnar* which go all the way down to the hands and provide the hands and fingers with their remarkable dexterity. Nerve disorders can result from injury or disease but the anatomy is so ingeniously constructed that such nerve problems are only seldom encountered in medical practice.

The elbow joint consists of three bones held together by strong ligaments and surrounding capsules. The upper arm bone (the humerus) comes down from the shoulder to the elbow joint to make contact with the forearm bones, the *radius* and *ulna,* at the elbow joint. It is so strong a union that fractures and dislocations are possible only when there is a fall or immense strain or trauma. Lubricated cartilages line the joint, making its operation smooth and easy.

For example, arthritis of the elbow is rather unusual compared to its frequency in other joints. Although the elbow is primarily a hinge, rotation of the head of the humerus makes inward and outward turns possible. Cushioning the back of the elbow is the *olecranon bursa,* sometimes a source of painful bursitis. Like the subdeltoid bursa, the olecranon bursa is a small sac that lies between the muscles, providing a cushioning effect and ease of function. "Tennis elbow" — a form of tendonitis — may be the result of prolonged and strenuous use.

The main arterial blood supply to the elbow comes from the *brachial* artery as it courses down the arm along the humerus. The front of the elbow is richer in blood vessels than the back. In front the brachial artery divides into large radial and ulnar branches but it also gives off several other branches that provide additional blood both to the back and the front of the elbow joint. Blood returns from the elbow and hand by way of the *antebrachial cephalic vein* which divides into the *brachial basilic vein* and the *brachial cephalic vein* as they jead towards the shoulder.

The main thing to remember is not the fancy names but the fact that the blood supply to the arm and shoulder is so good that injury through exercise or ordinary use is almost impossible. No maestro ever developed phlebitis from conducting an orchestra. No trapeze artist ever had to have an arm amputated because the circulation was blocked or even impaired. Whereas circulatory problems in the legs may be serious and even deadly, such disasters practically never occur in the arms.

While varicose veins in the legs are commonplace and indicative of some impairment in the venous return to the heart, varicose veins in the arms are practically nonexistent except in a few bizarre and extraordinary circumstances. In other words, even in the least active, nonathletic person, arm circulation is ordinarily excellent. Death from blood clots (embolism due to thrombophlebitis) from the arms is practically unknown. Clots that arise in the legs, break off, and land in the lungs are, unfortunately, still too common. Unlike leg joggers, arm joggers do not have the threat of disability—and even death—hanging over their heads.

Before going on to a discussion of the wrist and hands which are important to arm jogging too, mention must be made of the large muscles of the *thorax* (that part of the trunk between the neck and the abdomen) and the muscles of the neck that provide so much of the graceful, syncopated action of the arms and shoulders. Just as leg jogging needs the support of good muscles of the abdominal wall and lower abdomen, so do arm joggers need good musculature in the thorax and even in the neck.

In front of the thorax, under the breasts, are the

large *pectoral muscles,* both the *pectoralis major* and *pectoralis minor.* In back there are the *trapezius,* the *latissimus dorsi* muscles, the *teres major,* the *teres minor,* the *subscapularis* muscles and others. The *scalenus* muscles and the upper vertebral muscles help control the neck and the *deltoid* overrides the shoulder itself.

The intention in arm jogging is to develop these muscles for grace, efficiency and health, not merely for size and mass. It must be noted, however, that in weight lifting and other anaerobic exercises these same muscles of the arm, chest, neck and shoulder girdle can be developed to remarkable size and strength. To be a Mister America is not our goal. To emulate Charles Atlas or Arnold Schwarzenegger is not our goal. Unlike the remarkable longevity enjoyed by conductors of orchestras or members of championship rowing teams, there is no evidence that the "muscle-bound" athlete enjoys comparable longevity.

Aside from the fact that strengthening the pectoral muscles may in some young women improve breast size and in older women delay the onset of osteoporosis and prevent "dowager's hump," we urge arm exercises mostly for health and longevity, not for athletic prowess or beauty. We shall simply note here that there are more flat-chested ballerinas than trapeze artists. We shall also note that the women of the Caribbean who carry heavy baskets on their heads continue to stand erect even late in life. Spinal curvatures are rarely seen.

The anatomy of the hands and wrists (which can be considered as a single unit) is so complicated and miraculous as to defy any simple description. Hands are the primary instruments of toil, fabrication and artistry. Most of us earn our daily bread with our hands and depend on their manual dexterity for our very lives.

Hands are also prime instruments of communication, whether we "talk with our hands," beat tribal drums, flash semaphore signals, turn thumbs up or thumbs down, tap a telegraph key, or serve a brokerage house in the stock exchange pit.

Both the most primitive and the most sophisticated communications are accomplished through hand signals. Gestures of friendship, such as shaking hands, and gestures of contempt, such as thumbing one's nose, are hand signals.

Hands are also instruments of the fundamental issues of life — food, sex, behavior. We acquire food through hunting, fishing and agriculture. With our hands we throw stones, bait hooks, shoot arrows, pull triggers, gather rice. With our hands we cook and prepare foods to make them edible. We eat our food with fingers, forks, chopsticks; our cups and glasses are handheld. Hands are also instruments of sex, a fact that has gone largely unrecognized. Patting, fondling, hugging, caressing are almost entirely hand exercises. Making love without one's hands is almost inconceivable.

Hands are our primary instruments of aggressive behavior and hostility. The clenched fist is a universal signal of rebellion, anger and ferocity. The club, the lance, the sword, the slingshot, the machine gun, the dragger, the atomic bomb all are activated by hand action. Arms and hands are raised in a gesture of victory. Hands are held in supplication or in prayer.

No instrument devised by man matches the wizardry of human hands and fingers. The card sharp and the professional prestidigitator can use their fingers with such skill, speed and dexterity that their movements defy detection by the eye. The conductor of the Boston Symphony Orchestra, Seiji Ozawa, makes airy, graceful but-

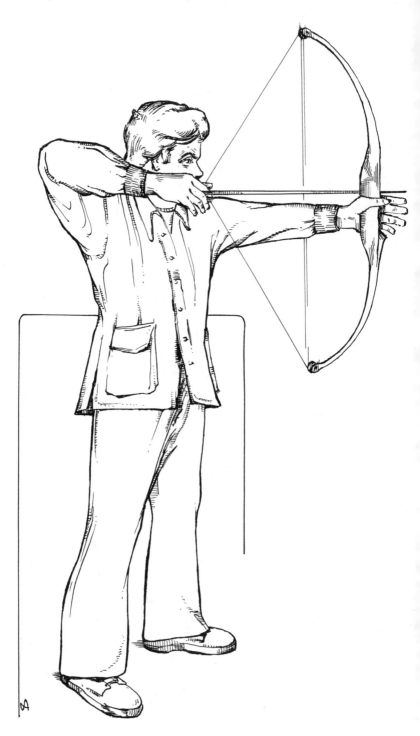

terfly patterns in the air with his left hand as he leads more forcefully with his right, describing images of visual beauty to accompany the auditory impact of the music. The finger cymbals of belly dancers heighten the wild, tempestuous rhythms of the dance. With a single sweep of the brush, the skilled calligrapher can describe beautiful patterns that evoke deep, primitive feelings in the observer. Almost without exception, all our art, all our clothing, all our literature, all our ornamentations is based on manual dexterity. It is not without good reason that *to be handy* is a term of approbation and *open-handedness* signifies candor, trust and sincerity.

With its multitude of bones, nerves, muscles, arteries, ligaments, tendons and veins, the hand provides us with the manual dexterity that distinguishes us from all other living creatures and, in an evolutionary sense, correlates with our brain size that exceeds that of even the largest of all the mammals. Over the millennia our hands have helped our brains grow and, reciprocally, our brains have added new dimensions to the skill with which we use our hands. No machine ever devised by man has yet come close to the hand's grace and perfection.

When comparisons are made between the legs and the arms, one striking observation is apparent — the distance between the heart and the fingers is much shorter than the distance between the heart and the toes. Even when both extremities are in the vertical distance position blood travels back and forth from the arm more easily than it does from the legs.

From the shoulder to the heart is a distance that one measures in inches; from the hips and thighs there may be several feet. Unless we are lying down, the veins in the legs are always working against a heavy gravitational load. In women, pregnancy places added stress on the circulation in the lower extremities. As we have already mentioned, varicose veins in the arms are exceedingly rare.

It is just because the hand-heart distance is shorter than the foot-heart distance and because the gravitational pull on the circulation of the arms is less than on the legs that arm jogging provides such immense advantages over running. Futhermore, since the arms are not weight-bearing they are less likely than the legs to be injured by exercise.

For most of us, whose lives are not completely sedentary, the legs get sufficient exercise in our daily routine. Ordinarily we walk enough each day to keep our leg muscles firm and healthy. Yet, unless we are orchestra leaders or house painters, hangers of acoustic tiles on ceilings, our arms never get enough exercise. The evidence is clear. For example, when swimming tires us out, the fatique is usually not in the legs but in the arms and thorax. The fatique of long sets of tennis is more often felt in the shoulder girdle than in the pelvis. Even the arms of professional boxers tire more easily than their legs.

Now that we understand the advantages of arm jogging and the need for arm exercise, let is direct our attention to those techniques that can enhance the arm skills that we need for better health and longer life.

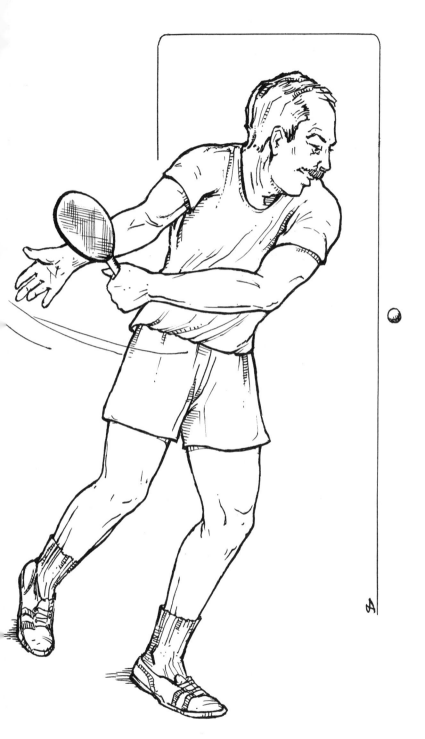

CHAPTER IV

Forgotten Functions of the Arms

Citizens of what state in the United States enjoy the greatest longevity and have the lowest incidence of illness and disability? Florida? California? Texas? Not at all! The answer is — *Vermont!*

Aside from the fact that Vermonters share the benefits of a hilly terrain (like their long-living counterparts in Turkestan, Switzerland and Tibet), Vermont is still primarily an agrarian state. Unless the statistics have been altered by the current influx of new residents, there are still more cows in Vermont than people. And it has to be pointed out that farmers and dairymen live active, vigorous lives.

Although there are many reasons why Vermonters live longer than the rest of us, one striking fact is that much of the daily work is done by hand in the hilly, rustic Vermont terrain. The vast mechanical reapers and harvesters of the flatlands of the Midwest are not as readily or as easily used in Vermont. The ox-drawn sled or wagon may move the stones and boulders from the farmland to the farm's boundaries but the loading and unloading of the stones and the fence-building are done primarily by hand. On smaller farms, too, hay be cut mechanically, but it is bundled and stored in the barns by hand. So at least one factor that promotes life and health in Vermont is strenuous *manual* labor.

During the past fifty years the amount of manual labor that we do has diminshed to such an extent that osteoporpsis of the neck bones and upper spine (in women, especially) has reached almost epidemic proportions. None of the solutions so far advanced by the medical profession has really helped or even made the slightest dent on the problem. Neither estrogens, calcium, fluorides, pulverized clam shells, chalk, vitamin D nor a host of other medicines work consistently or without hazard. The truth is that *what weakens bones most is disuse.*

What the doctors have failed to prescribe is hard arm work or arm and neck exercises. Osteoporosis could largely be *prevented* if arm, neck and shoulder exercises were started early enough in life. Isn't it strange that the giraffe who is forever using his long neck never develops osteoporosis or arthritis of the neck bone? Shouldn't this biologic fact have alerted the medical profession long ago?

With the loss of physical arm work or exercise has also come a concomitant loss in the stability of the institution of marriage. Skeptics may doubt this statement but the relationship between the two was described and defined for us many years ago by a leading female psychiatrist who shall be nameless. In the old days, this psychiatrist pointed out, the housewife who felt aggressive toward her husband could convert her hostility into action by beating a rug, scrubbing a floor, or hand-grating or chopping her carrots and cabbage. The modern housewife has few such physical outlets for her hostilities and the consequence is direct confrontation with her spouse. Although the reverse situation may also exist with the male unable to vent his aggressions or hostilities, physical outlets for the male are still more readily available. A man is more likely to hammer a board, hit a golf ball, change a flat tire, fling a frisbee.

Thus the advent of mechanical and electrical devices that do so much of our work for us has not only deprived us of the opportunity of improving our circulation, and strengthening the arms and bones of the neck, thorax and shoulders, but has also deprived us of the constructively aggressive use of our arms and hands.

Some of us can still remember how we chopped wood or shoveled coal into the furnace to stay warm in the winter. Automatic oil, gas or electric heat deprived us of this exercise. With oil now in short supply and expensive, the return to stoves that burn coal or wood may again provide us with a therapy that we had lost for half a century. One beneficial result of the oil shortage may be that it teaches us to use our arms and shoulders once again.

Prior to the advent of the vacuum cleaner, rugs were rolled up carried out to the back yard, draped over the clothesline or fence, and the dust was beaten out of them manually with a metal or wicker "rug-beater." It was hard work but there was satisfaction in seeing the dust fly and watching the bright colors return again to the fabric. And it was excellent exercise.

Similarly, scrubbing the floor with a bucket of warm

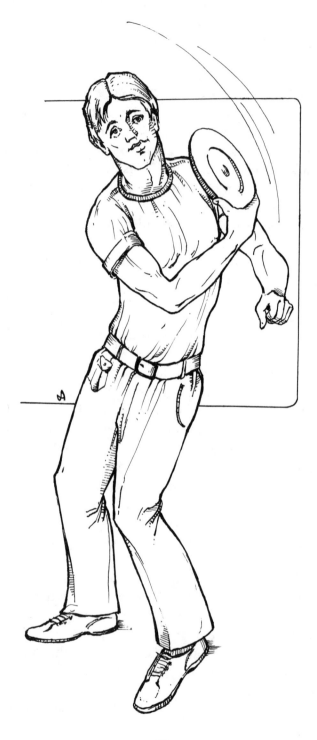

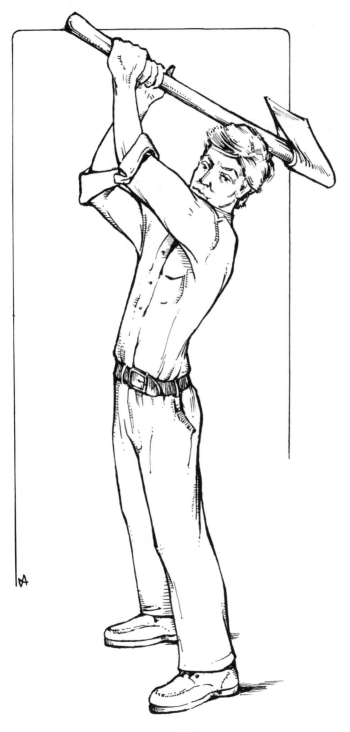

soapy water and a scrubbing brush was a job we all detested and tried to avoid. But when, in the past, there was no alternative mechanical cleaning method, we all got down on our knees and scrubbed away. Even today, those septuagenarian and octogenarians who still scrub their own kitchen floors are in far better physical shape than their contemporaries who have adopted easier methods. Scrubbing is a good, safe exercise for the arms, the shoulder girdle and the body as a whole.

Although many women all over the world still go down to the river and wash clothes by beating them on rocks or use a scrubbing board and a tub of water to get the clothes clean, most "industrialized" households either own a washing machine or are near a laundromat. Here again machines have brought about a reduction of "backbreaking" toil, but with the accompanying result of relieving the arms and back of beneficial exercise.

Some nameless male chauvinist has credited Charles Kettering's invention of the self-starter on automobiles as the initial step in the modern women's liberation movement. In the past, before one could ride, horses had to be saddled or automobiles had to be cranked. It took a lot of arm strength to crank a car, more strength than most women possessed. A woman had to have a man—a husband, a boyfriend, a hired chauffeur—or she stayed home, unliberated. The self-starter put women (and less powerful men) on wheels. But it also deprived men of arm exercise too.

There is no argument that mechanical devices are valuable. However, many of our work-saving machines and tools are paradoxically contributing to an increase in osteoporosis, a reduction in vigorous living, and a shortening of our potential life span. Our arms are definitely suffering from partial disuse atrophy and, if this continues, we may over the millennia lose our arms the way we lost our tail, our prehensile feet, or the ability to wiggle our ears effectively.

It has been a long time since our primitive ancestors swung from trees but it has also been a long time since we chopped wood, pulled bows, shot arrows, dug wells, sawed timber, yoked oxen, raised barns, built fortifications, painted ceilings, built stone viaducts, dueled with swords, or hauled water from a well. Most of us take full advantage of any and all labor-saving devices we can get our hands on. And then we simply sit at the bar, stagnate at the bridge table, drowse before the movie screen, or lounge in front of the one-eyed monster. Occasionally we move our hands to our face to eat or to wash. And that's all the exercise our arms get!

The deterioration of our arm muscles is likely to continue and perhaps even accelerate unless vigorous countermeasures are immediately taken. Should not there have been a clue to this problem centuries ago in the fact that Jesus himself was a *carpenter*? At any rate, we can do something *now* to correct this problem. First of all, we must recognize the fact that there *is* a problem and that it will not be solved by jogging. Our legs get enough exercise in our daily work; our arms and thorax are inadequately stressed! We must use our shoulders, our arms and our hands more. We *must*.

Since most of us will not discard our washing machines and return to scrubbing boards nor abandon the self-starters in our autos for the opportunity to crank the engine, and since few of us will chop our own wood to keep warm or knead bread dough, we must find other diversions and exercises to accomplish our goals.

While swimming, pitching horseshoes, and throwing

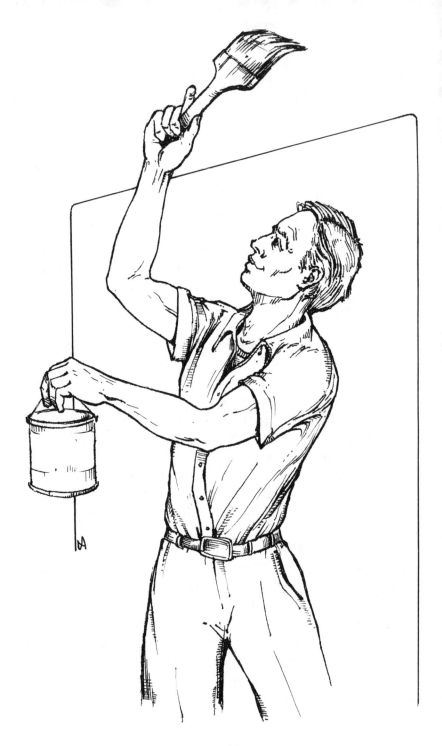

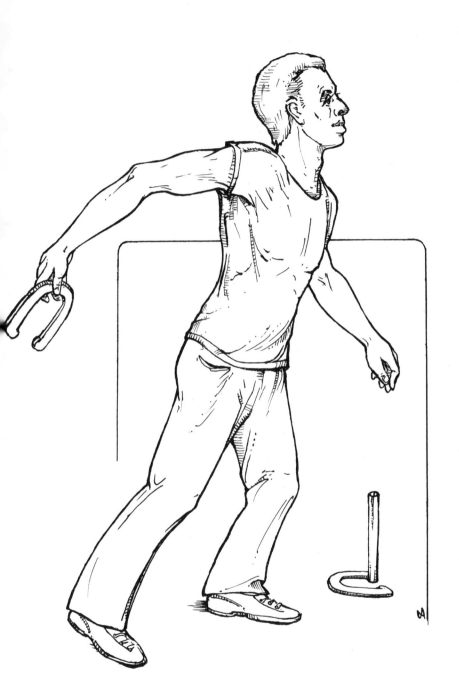

frisbees are great arm exercises, the opportunities for these sports are somewhat limited. Playing tennis is an excellent arm (and leg) exercise and is available to many. Perhaps the recent popularity of tennis has resulted from the recognition that so many other "arm" sports such as golf or billiards fail to provide enough arm exercise to make them really worthwhile. Also valuable are related sports such as handball, racquetball, volleyball, squash, lacrosse, and basketball. In almost every instance these arm sports provide exercise superior to jogging.

Bowling and such sports as curling, bocce and pitching horseshoes are unique because they provide excellent arm exercise at a slower pace than squash or tennis. Consequently these sports can be enjoyed by a wide range of ages, from childhood to the "golden years." An eight-year-old child can go bowling with his eighty-year-old grandmother! Grandpa can pitch horseshoes with his teenage grandson. Bocce, a quiet, old-world bowling game, has customarily been played by men, but more and more women are taking it up now.

Swimming of course is the sport *par excellence* for total arm and leg exercise. Backyard swimming pools are becoming more popular as the prices of gasoline and travel rise. However, in temperate climates, outdoor swimming is available for only two or three months so its value as an exercise is limited. Where indoor community swimming pools or YMCA pools are available, they should be taken full advantage.

While ordinary ballroom dancing provides some exercise, disco, flamenco, chassidic, square dancing and other ethnic dances make you use your arms as well as your legs. It was jitterbug and rock-and-roll that taught American youth over a generation ago that dancing was more enjoyable when the arms went into action as well as

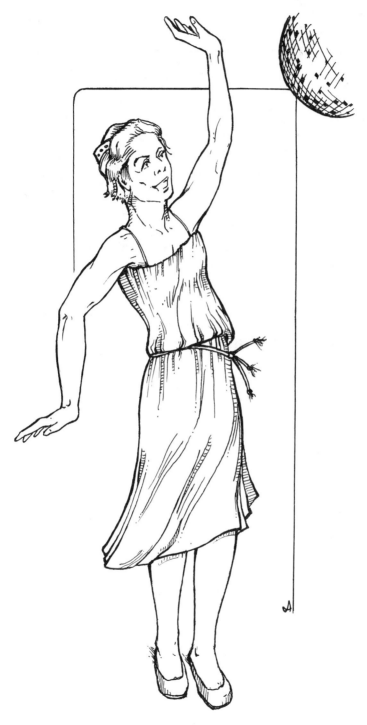

the legs. Although disco dancing today is the subject of some criticism by touch-dancers, it must be pointed out that disco dancers use their arms almost as much as their legs. There is no doubt that disco provides more exercise than circling to a Vienese waltz or drowsing with your partner on the dance floor to a Lawrence Welk foxtrot.

Something else this generation has forgotten is how to row, how to pull vigorously on the ears. We have also forgotten how therapeutic this exercise can be. Recently the magazine *Modern Maturity* reported on Stan Mullin, a sixty-eight-year-old Los Angeles lawyer who had fractured his pelvic bone and could no longer ride his ten-speed bike.

It was only after he returned to his forty-fifth reunion at Harvard that he was reminded of the times he had spent sculling on the Charles River. He was inspired to try again the sport that had once given him such pleasure.

Today he works out four times a week, sculling in the Pacific Ocean for four miles in his twenty-seven-pound racing shell. Stan Mullin's physician, Dr. John Sack, says this about sculling:

> "I've recommended sculling to many older people looking for a sport that offers all-around conditioning. Sculling can fit that bill; it's a sport with no age barriers.
>
> Because the rower is seated while exercising and doesn't carry his body weight, the overall effect on the body is more calming than, say jogging or tennis.
>
> "There is less agitation; you don't have the shock to the body that other sports can give you, the constant pounding of the joints. Whether you decide to take it easy or beat yourself into the ground,

you're not going to hurt yourself. Basically, when you get through, you'll just be good and tired."[1]

Yet the most remarkable advantages of arm exercising is that it can easily be a private, personal performance. Unlike jogging, you don't need an outdoor track, a road or highway or an indoor arena. You don't need a swimming pool or a tennis court. You need only the space your own body ocupies. You can exercise your arms while lying on your back or rolled over for push-ups. You can sit on a chair or stand up. You can even do handstands.

Arm exercising is possible under almost any circumstances with almost no limitations of time or space. All that is necessary is the recognition of the value and importance of arm exercises. All that is necessary is twenty to thirty minutes twice a day. Arm exercises can be done to music or in complete silence. They can be done singly, in pairs, or in groups. They require no special equipment or they can be done with backyard "jungle-gyms," special parallel bars, or even costly trapezes. They can be done empty-handed or with batons or wooden weighted dumbbells. The possibilities are endless.

---

[1]Suzanne Murphy, "Stan Mullin's Flying Oars," *Modern Maturity,* August-September 1979, p. 12.

CHAPTER V

Arm Exercises for Beginners

On a quiet beach in Nantucket last summer we saw four preteen girls playing a game that should serve them well even later in life. One, the leader, watched the three others and counted as they attempted to do handstands. The leader replaced the youngster who stayed up the longest and the players rotated from leader to follower all during the afternoon. At an early age these youngsters were learning an important lesson — how to use their arms and their thoracic muscles to great advantage.

Watching these girls, we were reminded of an incident at our office some years ago when we congratulated a descendant of the Vikings because our examination showed that he was in excellent health. He smiled and said, "I thought I was." Then he explained. "Last year at my seventy-fifty birthday party my guests began ribbing me about my old age. So I did a handstand, walked around the room on my hands, and shook hands with each of the guests."

Then, before our eyes and to our great surprise, this patient did a handstand in our consultation room and walked around the entire room on his hands to show us that he still had the strength and stamina and the *youth*. When he was younger, he said, he had been a circus acrobat. Now, although he had been retired for almost twenty years, he continued the exercises that had been the source of his strength and endurance.

But we are getting ahead of our exercise program. Most of our readers and patients are neither circus acrobats nor in training to become Olympic stars. Most of us cannot do handstands, nor should we even attempt them. Most of us should start with a *simple* exercise program. And be sure to consult your own doctor before starting this or *any* exercise plan.

An almost infallibly safe way to start arm exercising is by lying on your back on the carpeted floor. This is the best approach for any age group and especially for senior citizens. By lying on the floor a minimal amount of strain is placed on the heart and the circulation system doesn't have to fight the untoward effects of gravity. A small pillow placed under the head will make the exercises even easier.

Begin by lying flat on your back and extending your arms fully over your head. At first you may feel a little strain in your back and shoulder blades as the muscles stretch out but the effort is well worth it. Bring your arms forward to your sides, describing an upward arc of 180% as you do so. Set your own pace. Try for ten arm raises at first, and gradually work up to twenty or thirty.

Although simple exercise such as this can be carried out in silence on your bedroom floor, you will probably

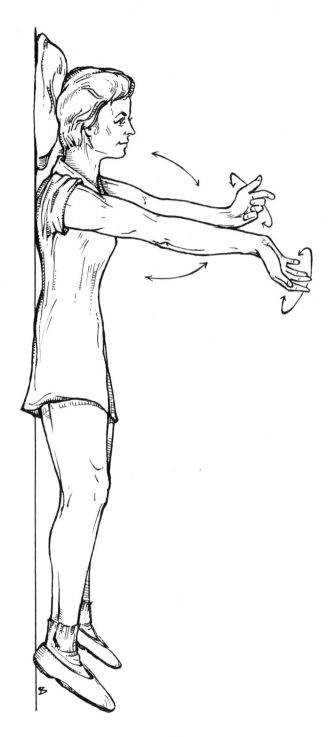

enjoy your exercises more with music. An inexpensive portable AM-FM transistor radio is fine or if you have a tape recorder and your own favorite tapes, that's even better. Use the music you like and the rhythm that suits you. Remember — *you* determine the *speed* of your exercises. You can move your arms in time to a slow, classical symphony or to an ear-splitting disco beat. That is one of the great advantages arm exercises have over leg exercises — you can move your arms slower or faster than your legs.

By playing a given musical selection (or selections) over and over again, you will develop an exercising rhythm that you enjoy. Later on, when you do your exercises standing up, you can be the conductor of your own symphony orchestra. All of us have enough recessive Walter Mitty chromosomes to call upon when we want to perform like Arturo Toscanini or like John Philip Sousa. It's even more fun if you conduct your imaginary orchestra facing a mirror!

⬤ A second exercise you can easily do while lying down is "punching the air" above you or, if you prefer, imagine turning a bicycle wheel with your outstretched arm. This, our second exercise, is considerably more tiring than our first and should be pursued only intermittently with short rest periods in between. Rolling over and doing push-ups is even more strenuous and should not be undertaken by the older novice since, with push-ups, you are working against gravity. This, like jogging, may strain the heart and the chest muscles.

Since arm exercises can be carried out in both the lying and sitting positions, they are excellent for people who are semi-ambulatory or bedridden. Even for those who are not disabled, a smart idea is to start your arm exercises first thing in the morning sitting at the edge of the bed. Brain circulation and arm circulation are closely

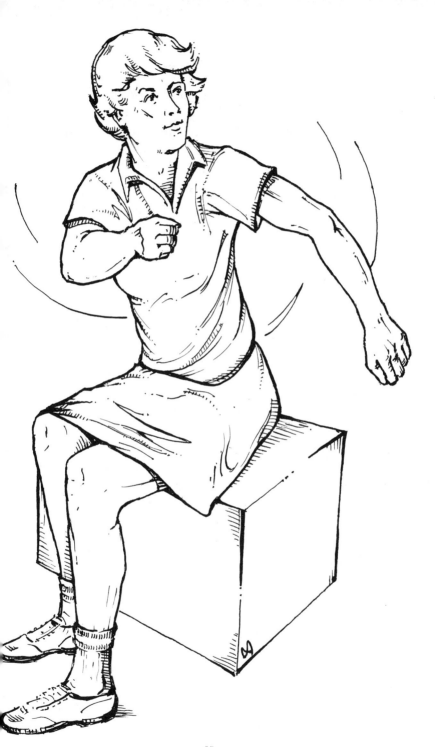

related. The arteries to both the arms and the brain are branches off the upper aorta as it leaves the heart. Even wiggling your fingers or flapping your arms or wrists will speed circulation to the brain. The dull, stupid, depressed feeling of the night will quickly disappear and you will feel more alert and ready to go. Have your morning coffee *after* your morning arm exercises and you will even find the coffee more enjoyable. For most people, arm exercises are an effective method of preventing usual morning grouchiness.

An ordinary rubber ball is another simple device for exercising the arms. A ball can be bounced off the floor, off a wall, or thrown up in the air and caught. We can play catch by ourselves or with a friend, a neighbor, a child or a grandchild. It's sad but most of us have forgotten how to play catch. We should learn again. It's good exercise. And good fun.

In European health spas many years ago physicians learned about the therapeutic value of throwing a heavier ball around — the "medicine" ball. Participants in the game stood in a circle and the ball, about the size of a basketball, was thrown from one player to another in a regular or in a hapharzard fashion. Doctors, over fifty years ago, found this useful in helping patients recover from tuberculosis and, more recently, for speeding recovery from heart attacks. In this exercise the patient stands almost fixed in one spot, his legs spread slightly apart to steady his balance, and the arms and torso are moved to catch or throw the ball. The game continues for a half-hour or longer or until the participants are tired.

Heaving the medicine ball back and forth is something that we recommend to our patients, especially during the recovery phase of an illness or an injury. It can be undertaken as soon as the patient can get out of bed, and

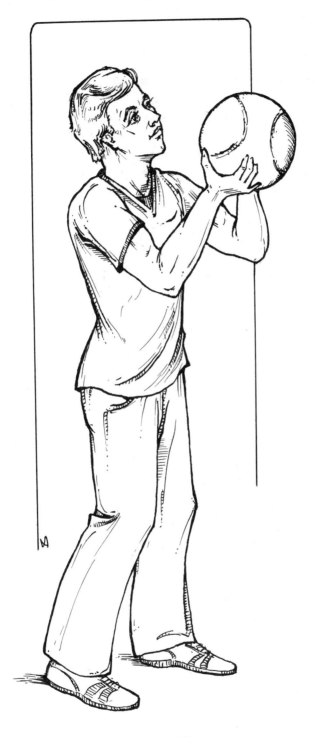

can even be played from a wheel chair. It is a pity that this exercise, with a long tradition of success behind it, has been ignored by American physicians or replaced by stress testing, walking on costly automated ramps. Compared to almost any kind of leg exercise, especially jogging, throwing a medicine ball is more exercise and less stress. It is both healthier and safer.

Once you are up on your feet, the arm exercises that you can enjoy are almost endless. And new discoveries about their health value are being made all the time. Take, for example, Raynaud's syndrome, a painful affliction in which there is blanching of the finger tips (and sometimes, in advanced cases, *gangrene*) due to spasm of the small arteries of the hands and wrists. Yet is was just recently discovered that swinging your arms as if you were pitching a softball underhand improves the circulation to the fingers and relieves the blanching and pain.

You don't have to have Raynaud's syndrome to exercise each arm like a softball pitcher. Try it now, ten times each arm. Pause and rest for a minute. Try it ten times again. You can feel the warmth in your arms, your face and in your chest. Repeat the exercise two or three (or more) times a day if you wish. Try it in the morning to wake you up. Try it at night to help you sleep better.

Notice how a cat stretches its forepaws after resting or when it wakes up. This is such a natural and beneficial thing to do. Yawn and stretch! It's an easy way to revitalize yourself. The Japanese have taken advantage of this simple exercise to increase industrial productivity. In many of their factories periods of intense work are broken up by exercise. No jogging! The Japanese workers extend their arms, rotate their arms, and stretch their torsos. These exercises are done in unison, all the workers following a set pattern. Stretch and twist. Stretch and

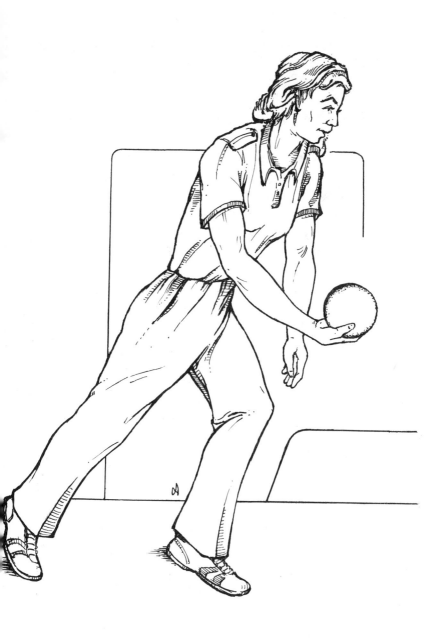

twist. Then they can resume work considerably relaxed and refreshed. Is it any wonder that Japan has enjoyed a postwar economic miracle while we keep jogging backward into a recession? Productivity depends on efficient use of *hands* and *brains,* not legs and buttocks. Arm exercises should be *mandatory* for our factory workers and others who work in production or assembly lines.

Arm exercises should be started in childhood or as early in life as possible. A person is never too young (or too old) to begin. For good posture and a straight back later in life, you must start exercising your arms and torso at an early age. The youngster who does chin-ups, shoots baskets, climbs trees and swims will have better posture and a straighter spine than one who neglects such physical activities. Indeed, many years ago, freshmen students entering Harvard were checked for their posture and had a full silhouette of their frame photographed on a grid. Those freshmen who failed to meet Harvard's posture standards were required to take a program of setting-up exercises to strengthen their arms and back. Later they were checked again and the degree of improvement was noted on their records.

Now let's all stand up and do some simple arm exercises in a relaxed standing position.

✳️Get your arms up and away from your sides and hold them outstretched like a bird flying. Flex your elbows and flex your wrists and gently flap your arms about for a while like a bird. Now straighten your arms again, put them up straight above your head and clap your hands over your head. Repeat this fifteen or twenty times. Now with arms outstretched, clap your hands in front of you twenty times. Now rest.

Put your arms up and out again and roll your outstretched arms in their sockets. Rotate your arms twenty times clockwise and twenty times counterclock-wise. Rest again. Finally, the beginner can spend a few minutes of his upright exercise time pretending to be vigorously punching a bag (or some other object or person), conducting a symphony orchestra, or sparring with some unseen partner. Remember during all these exercises that the beginner *should take it easy*. These exercises are designed to stimulate circulation and improve health. They are *not* designed to make you a professional fighter or weight lifter. Indeed, one of the things we want to avoid is the muscle-bound, hypertrophied muscular form of the weight lifter. We want our muscles supple like those of the carpenter, tennis player, flamenco dancer. Never allow yourself to get too tired or too short of breath.

At first you can time yourself, spending about ten minutes morning and night on your exercises. Later, as you become more proficient, you will be able to determine by the timer "in your bones" about how much exercise is enough for you.

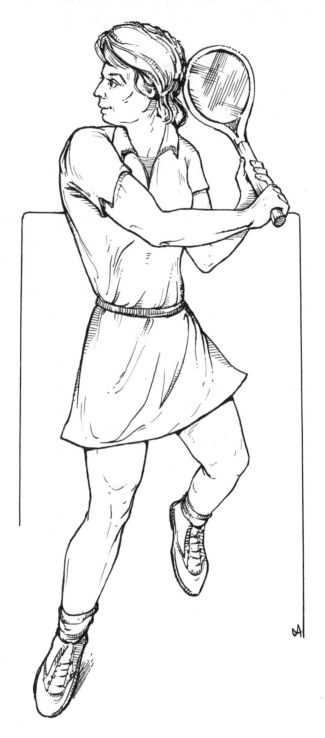

CHAPTER VI

Arm Exercises
for the More Proficient

After a few weeks of simple arm exercises, you still may not be able to do handstands or throw a javelin fifty yards, but you should find it much easier to hang the drapes, wash the kitchen walls, or paint the side of the barn. Besides, you will be enjoying a better, all-over sense of well-being. Even holding a hand at bridge as you sit around the card table or pushing the cart at the supermarket will be easier.

In most people, the leg muscles are already strong enough because they *work against a resistance*. They usually need no further strengthening unless for a specific purpose such as a sport or a job. Leg muscles support the shifting weight of the body, moving as they do against

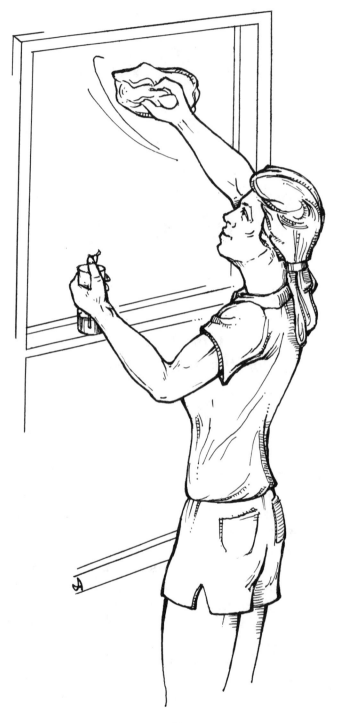

gravitational forces. One can easily appreciate the difference between the muscular development of the arms and the legs by looking, for example, at the kangaroo or the jack rabbit. Limbs that are used for locomotion and weight bearing are much heavier and stronger than the forepaws. Not only are the bones stronger and heavier but the muscles that move them are also increased in size and strength.

And this is the most important clue to muscular power and energy — *muscles get stronger as they work against resistance.* Bones also share in this unique ability to waste away when they are not used and to strengthen with exercise, *expecially resistance.*

Years ago when patients with tuberculosis of the spine were treated by prolonged rest in a plaster body cast that extended from the armpits to the knees, doctors observed that many of the patients developed painful calcium kidney stones. The bones of the tuberculosis victims softened as they remained in their casts and the calcium lost from the bones passed into the kidneys and formed the agonizing stones there.

Then doctors learned to turn the patients over two or three times each day so that part of the time the patients lay on their backs and at other times on their stomachs. In many cases, calcium loss could be prevented by simply rotating the patient as he lay in his plaster cast.

Since tuberculosis of the spine is a rare disorder nowadays, most doctors have forgotten the valuable lesson learned a generation or more ago. Immobility wastes both muscles and bones. Prolonged inactivity wastes both muscles and bones. On the contrary, physical activity strengthens both muscles and bones. Orthopedists know that the quickest way to rehabilitate a patient after a bone injury or bone surgery is to start an exercise program as soon as possible. Yet both orthopedists and internists have so far failed to recognize the importance of exercise in preventing osteoporosis.

Since osteoporosis is more common in women than in men and since it is especially disabling when it weakens the bones of the neck and upper thorax, arm exercises must be started early in life to prevent calcium loss and wasting. Once the neck bones are weakened and collapsed, exercise cannot restore normal structure or function although it may prevent further damage. While the exercises described in the previous chapter may be helpful, they do not provide adequate stress. And it must be emphasized that it is *stress* that really strengthens the bones and muscles.

One simple technique for stressing the arms and shoulders requires two inexpensive items that can be purchased in your local hardware store — a clothesline pulley and a few feet of clothesline rope. The pulley is screwed into the top of an infrequently used door opening and a length of clothesline, about four or five feet, is threaded through the pulley.

Sit comfortably on a chair in the doorway opening and grasp the loops that have been knotted at the ends of the clothesline. Then, as the right arm pulls down, pull up with the left arm. The movement is the normal reciprocal action that one experiences in walking or crawl-swimming. The gravitational weight of one arm provides the resistance for the other arm.

While this exercise is especially valuable for people who may have a limited range of shoulder motion after an injury or an attack of tendonitis, it is also of great value to anyone who wants to keep his shoulders strong and the chest and shoulder muscles supple and limber.

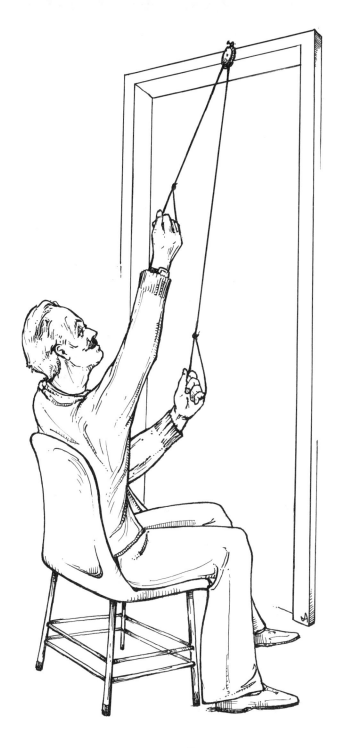

Two clothesline pulleys and clothesline cord can provide the arms and thorax with a vigorous, healthy workout. The pulleys can be screwed against the wall in the bedroom or in the cellar about twelve to eighteen inches apart from each other and about five or six feet off the floor. Pass a clothesline cord through each pulley and knot the end that you grasp for easy holding. The other end can be tied on to some suitable weights such as old steam irons or even large, empty juice cans filled with sand or rocks. A snip of wire from a coat hanger can be used to fasten the cans to the rope. If empty juice cans are used as weights, start with them half-filled and gradually increase the weights as the muscles get stronger.

For this exercise, you can stand either facing the wall or with the back turned to the wall. It is easier to start facing the wall. Grasp a knotted end of the cord with each hand and pull toward you away from the wall. Pulling the weights with each arm fifteen or twenty times is a good way to start. This exercise can be repeated two or three times a day. This device costs you practically nothing yet is as effective in building muscles as anything found in costly health spas.

Furthermore, you are master all the time of your creation. You can change the weights at will. You don't have to pay dues to any health club. You can exercise at hours that are convenient to you. Exercising can keep you warmer in the winter. You don't have to waste gasoline and money to have this simple "health spa" in your own home. Working with music (a transistor radio or a tape recorder) can make the exercises even more fun.

Stressing your arms and shoulder muscles can also be accomplished through the use of a simple overhead bar. The simplest bar can be fixed across the top of a slightly used closet or a doorway, fastened permanently

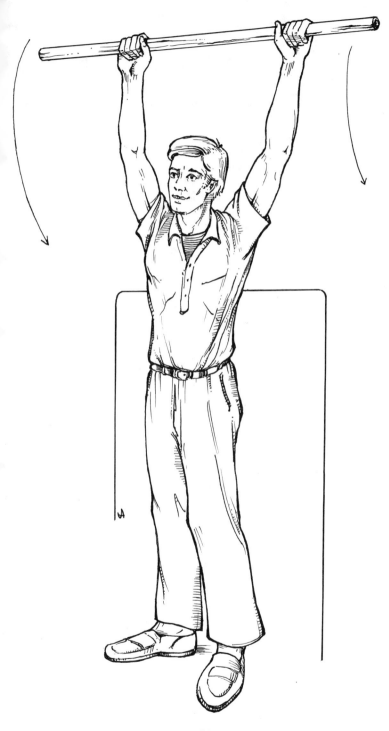

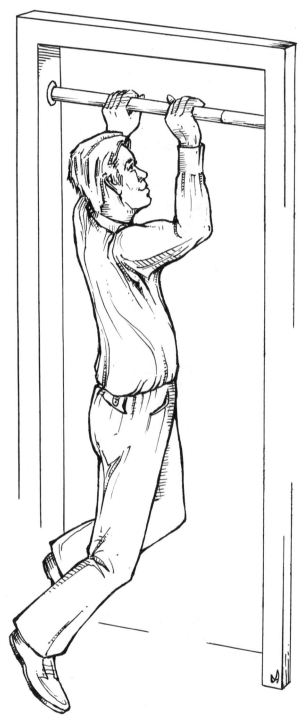

or placed in a wooden slot so it can be removed when not in use. Even if your muscles are not strong enough to chin yourself on the bar, the bar can still be used to raise your body off the floor.

This is not an exercise for the novice. It takes a great deal of muscular effort to pull your own weight up. Still, pulling against the bar is a worthwhile effort even if you raise yourself only momentarily, only an inch or two off the floor.

Parallel bars are far more complicated than the single bar suspended in a doorway. For parallel bars you must have lots of room and the bars should be firmly suspended from a ceiling. Special bolts and connectors may be necessary to keep them firmly in place. A garage or a cellar might be a suitable area. Parallel bars can be used the way a youngster uses an outdoor jungle gym, moving along them off the floor, grabbing each bar as you move along. This is a vigorous exercise since your arms are being used to move your entire body several inches off the floor.

If you live in a small apartment or are not handy, you can dispense with ropes and pulleys. Extra weights can be hand held. Holding a couple of old, heavy shoes in each hand will give you added resistance. Or you can stitch lead weights into an old pair of gardening gloves. A short length of metal bar can be used as a baton and brought forward to an overhead position. Professional weighted and balanced dumbbells can be carefully swung around over your head.

Unlike jogging where the exercise is uniform and monotonous (unless you are chased by a dog), the variety of arm exercises that you can enjoy is endless. You can be as inventive as you wish. Even throwing darts at a board is good exercise and good fun. If you have the space for it, you might try climbing a twelve-foot pole. Skipping rope gives exercise to both your arms and legs.

Try breaking up your heavy exercises with a spell of lighter ones. An easy exercise commonly used by orthopedic specialists to limber up a "frozen" shoulder joint is to have the patient stand about two feet away from a wall, lean forward with both outstretched arms, and use both hands to "climb" upward on the wall as high as possible. This stretches both shoulders to their maximum range and enhances mobility. This exercise can be repeated as many times as you wish. It is 100 percent safe and effective.

A second simple orthopedic exercise for improving shoulder function is to lean forward on a table with one hand while the other free arm droops over the table's edge. Rotate the free arm easily in an arc, around and around, both clockwise and counterclockwise, for maximum range and flexibility. Then reverse hands. If shoulder adhesions are present, they can be loosened by this exercise. It is almost impossible to get tired out by doing this, no matter how often you do it.

Although walking around balancing a load of books on your head is not strictly an arm exercise, it is valuable in bringing added control to the back and shoulder muscles. Even though you may never acquire the skill of a Caribbean housewife who brings all her shopping home in a head basket, walking around with a stack of books on your head is still good for your posture and balance. You can even make believe that it is a diamond tiara you are wearing and not a pile of books. The one-book load that you should start with can be later increased to three or four books. The heavier the weight your neck supports, the stronger your bones and muscles will become.

When you are ready to try something more difficult

after carrying out the arm exercises described in these chapters, you can move on to the "tripod." This further strengthens your neck and shoulders and should be done on the floor. Lying on your back, stretch your legs out straight and spread your feet about ten to twelve inches apart. Now push down at the same time with the back of your skull and with your heels and try to make a tripod out of your (straight) body. You should be touching the floor with only your head and heels. Try to lift your whole body off the floor with this maneuver. This is not easy to do, but even if you can't complete it, just working at it for a few minutes a day will make your back and neck stronger. The "tripod" is *not* an exercise for the novice or beginner however, so don't attempt it unless you have your doctor's permission or are in excellent physical condition.

Although isometric exercises are less effective than those conducted through a range of motion, they are still better than no exercises at all. Besides, isometrics have the advantage of taking up no space and requiring no special equipment. Try, for example, standing in a wide doorway and pushing both sides of the doorway away from you. The doorway will not move (unless you have the strength of Sampson) but the muscles of your arms will be stressed.

Grasp your hands in front of you, locking one palm against the other. Now, keeping your fingers firmly flexed, try to pull one hand away from the other. Keep your hands tightly clenched and try pulling your arms apart. Repeat as often as you like. You can practice these exercises while watching television or even in a movie theater.

Remember, we must move and exercise our arms more if we wish to enjoy the best possible health. Labor-saving devices like the powered chainsaw, the vacuum cleaner and the paint spray gun have eased our lives but have made our muscles weak and our bones osteoporotic. We must learn again to work more physically with our arms and shoulders or we must exercise. Anything less leads certainly to disability and impairment of vigor.

CHAPTER VII

Almost Anyone Can JARM

Mike O'Brien was a bit "hard of hearing" but that was his *only* physical impairment. For over ten years he had been coming to our office for annual check-ups and he was always found to be in excellent health. Three years ago, at the age of eighty-five, he had to give up playing handball because it was getting too strenuous.

"But I still get plenty of exercise," said Mike.

"What do you do now?" I asked.

"I stretch out my arms like this and I roll my arms around forty times like this and then forty times in the opposite direction," Mike said as he demonstrated these exercises. He went on to lie on the office floor to show us how he "rides" an imaginary inverted bicycle while on his back.

He continued to describe and show us his whole

series of exercises for almost five minutes. Even with what seemed like a great deal of exertion for an older man, Mike never appeared short of breath or winded. All his life he had been intuitively wise enough to exercise his arms as well as hig legs. In his youth he had been in the merchant marine and had worked part time as a stevedore. He had always exercised his arms. Handball was the sport he enjoyed most, even into his eighties.

Before we encourage everyone to swing his arms vigorously to and fro or up and down, we must add one *note of caution:*

DO NOT EXERCISE YOUR ARMS VIGOROUSLY IF YOU FEEL FAINT, GET LIGHTHEADED, HAVE HEAD PAIN, OR WEAKNESS OR PARALYSIS IN AN ARM.

Doctors know that in some *unusual* circumstances, exercising the arms may actually deprive the brain of blood and thus induce weakness, faintness or any of the other symptoms noted above. This phenomenon is known as the subclavian steal and was first described in 1961 in the *New England Journal of Medicine* by Dr. Martin Reivich and his associates at the University of Pennsylvania School of Medicine.

While arm exercises almost always improve blood flow to the brain, such exercises can, *under some very unusual circumstances,* siphon blood from the brain. To understand how this happens one needs to review the anatomy of the blood vessels that come off the heart.

The *aorta* is the main artery. The main branch going to the right is the *innominate artery.* Short in length, it divides quickly into an upper branch, the *common carotid artery* that goes upward to the head and brain and to another branch, the *right subclavian artery* behind the collarbone) that goes to the right arm. Further along on the right of the subclavian artery is the *right vertebral artery,* another blood vessel that goes to the brain via the bones in the back of the neck.

On the left, off the aorta, the first (and upward) branch is the left *common carotid artery.* Like its right counterpart, this artery carries blood to the head and the brain. The second branch off the aorta on the left is the *left subclavian artery* which goes directly to the left arm. Just a little beyond this point, leading off the left subclavian artery, is the *left vertebral artery* that follows the same course as its partner on the right.

Ultimately both vertebral arteries meet and hook up in the brain to form the *basilar artery* which, after additional branches and turns, joins the other branches from the carotid artery coming up to the head from the front of the neck (*carotids*) and those in the back of the spine (the vertebrals).

Now here is the problem. If the left subclavian artery is partially blocked by a clot or some narrowing just before the point where the vertebral artery starts to take off, any increased arm movement, or even some neck motions, creates a suction effect in the left vertebral artery so that blood is sucked away (*or stolen*) from the brain. That's why this problem is called the subclavian steal. Although it's rare (only a dozen cases have been reported in the medical literature), you should be aware that such a condition can exist.

But let us repeat. If you have any symptoms such as *weakness, dizziness, head pain* or *disturbances in vision,* you should *not* continue your arm exercises and you should *see your doctor.*

Another medical problem that arm joggers may encounter is circulatory in a sense but not quite as serious. It's called thoracic outlet syndrome.

That part of the thorax where the arm joins the chest is known technically as the *thoracic outlet*. Important nerves, blood vessels and other structures are all compressed anatomically here into narrow quarters, most of them behind the collar bone.

The main arteries to the arms, the subclavian arteries, lie (as we have already noted) behind the collarbone. These arteries, right and left, also lie just a bit in front of the first rib. In some people this area is so tight that some muscles and ribs compress or squeeze the subclavian arteries so tightly that blood flow to the arms and hands is reduced. The motion most likely to compress the arteries is elevation of the arm above the head.

Ordinary arm exercises should cause only the *normal* fatigue that comes with any exertion. But if arm exercises make your fingers numb or cause you to drop things from your hand, you may have thoracic outlet syndrome and you should consult your doctor.

A third possible problem is the carpal tunnel syndrome. This is a wrist disorder but it can be mistaken for a pinched nerve in the neck or a variant of the thoracic outlet syndrome. Patients with this disorder suffer from numbness or tingling or pain in the hand (or hands) which is worse when using the hands for activities requiring wrist action such as driving, sewing or using wrenches. If the pain awakens the patient at night (a common problem), the patient invariably tries to relieve his distress by shaking or rubbing his hand, hanging it over the side of the bed, or running hot or cold water on the hand.

This disorder is called carpal tunnel syndrome because there is a "tunnel" under the carpal (wrist) ligament through which passes a large nerve (the median) to the thumb and first three fingers of the hand. Sufferers from carpal tunnel syndrome are usually not helped by medicine. Cortisone injections into the wrist help only temporarily. The main problem is that the carpal tendon is too tight across the wrist and the median nerve is thus bound down and compressed. Surgery gives prompt, and sometimes almost miraculous, cures. When a surgeon operates, he cuts the tendon and looses the nerve.

Patients often ask about what kind of exercises they can do in the shower or in the tub. Invariably we discourage such activities. It is too easy to slip in the shower or bang your hands against the wall of the tub. It is far better to exercise *before* bathing and then soak in the refreshing warmth of the water after the *jarming* is finished.

There is one great exercise, however, that can be taken in water especially if the water is comfortably warm. That exercise is swimming.

One of my patients owned a seaside summer home for twenty years but he had never gone into the ocean because the water (north of Cape Cod) was simply too cold. However, when he saw a notice in his newspaper that he could swim in his local YMCA's *heated* pool, he thought that was a great idea and joined the Y.

All across the country there are many organizations that offer pool memberships and even have special rates for older people. Some hotels and motels allow "outsiders" to use their pools for a nominal annual fee. Many of our patients are thus able to swim all year round.

Unlike golf, swimming is an ideal sport for most persons, even older ones, because it is noncompetitive. Except in racing meets, the swimmer competes only against himself. While the golfer is often a saddened and disgruntled person (on the twelfth hole he sliced the ball into the woods), the swimmer luxuriates in pure joy. He

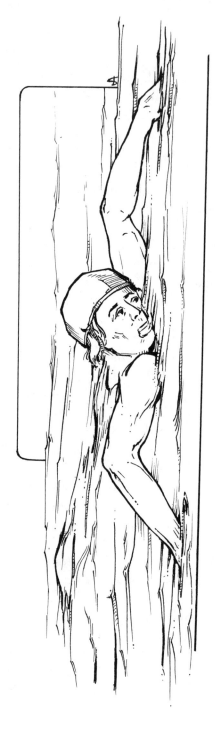

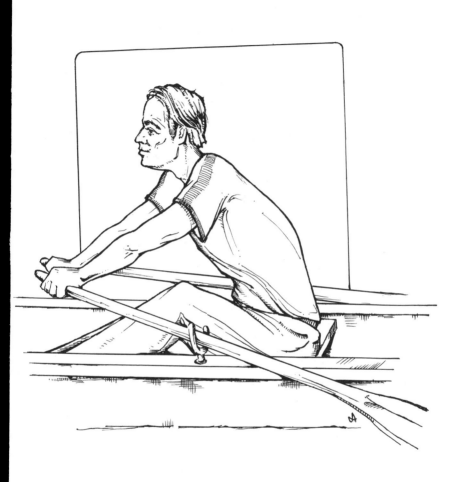

83

is almost always master of his own destiny, starting and stopping when he wishes and swimming those strokes that provide pleasure. Besides, along with swimming, additional exercises can be performed in the water or at poolside.

Doc Counsilman, the oldest person (at fifty-eight) to swim the English Channel and the former trainer of Olympic star Mark Spitz, advises senior citizens to start swimming gradually and work up to a comfortable pace that has them breathing heavier than usual but not in a labored way. He also is a believer in kicking drills using a swimboard, goggles and "warming down" after a swim. "Just set your own pace," he says. Swim relaxed and feel good.

Of course arm exercise is provided also by simple chores and household jobs. Washing your own car and even waxing it provide good arm exercise (and the pleasant experience of seeing your happy face reflected in the shine) and will save you many dollars.

You can also abandon the electric hedge clippers. Electricity costs too much now. Besides, the electric clipper can destroy fingers or, if improperly insulated and grounded, can cause nasty shocks. A hedge trimmed by hand can be true artistry as well as healthy arm exercise.

There is hardly a chore around the house that can't be re-evaluated from the standpoint of beneficial arm exercise, as well as in terms of reducing costs by saving electricity. You can scrub pots and pans instead of putting them in the dishwasher. You can wash, wring out, and hang your laundry instead of using the washer/dryer. You can use a carpet sweeper instead of a vacuum cleaner on the rugs. Just look around and you'll see many other household activities that can be tranformed into beneficial exercise that is economical too.

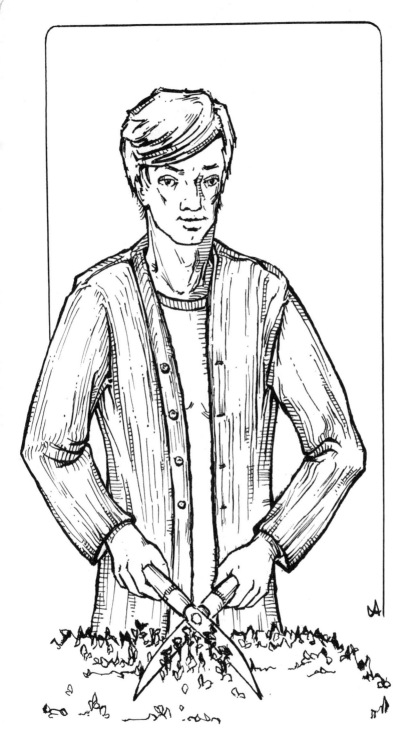

Arm exercises can easily be merged with other activities involving the trunk, the neck and the rest of the body. Skipping rope, for example, combines both arm and leg exercises into a synthesis of grace and beauty. Just how effectively one can use such torso-and-arm exercises can be illustrated by the following personal experience.

Some years ago, in my beachfront hotel room in Tel Aviv, I was awakened shortly before six in the morning by noises that drifted in through the window. People were talking on the beach, making muffled rhythmic sounds, clapping their hands. When I looked out at the beach I saw eleven tow-headed people, Swedish tourists I had met the previous evening, all doing early morning calisthenics. Some, in small groups, were doing a common exercise in unison, others improvised on their own. In addition to some of the simple arm exercises described in the previous chapter, they combined arm-and-torso exercises with amazing grace and skill.

In one exercise, for example, they bent forward and repeatedly touched the toes of the right foot with the fingers of the left hand. Then they reversed the procedure and touched the toes of the left foot with the fingers of the right hand. They continued this exercise for about five minutes.

Then they switched to a more difficult variation. They leaned far backwards, touching first the left heel with the tips of the fingers of the right hand, then the right heel with the left hand. They repeated this exercise about twenty times.

I watched in fascination for about twenty minutes. Is there any wonder, I thought, that the Swedes are among the healthiest people in the world? And probably the most beautiful.

The value of arm exercises has alredy been recognized and appreciated in some nursing homes were geriatric patients are truly limited in the range and scope of their activities. Recently we made a nursing home call to see an eighty-two-year-old patient. Only four months earlier, when she was first admitted, she had complained bitterly that she had been cast aside by her family, that she had been put into the nursing home against her will. Now, a few months later, she was all smiles.

"I just bowled a strike," she grinned. "I'm the captain of my team."

She explained that the bowling alley in the nursing home was smaller than regulation size and the bowling balls were lighter. Yet she bowled three days a week —and enjoyed every minute of it.

In other nursing homes which we visit we often see a group leader clap hands and sing songs while her geriatric chorus (usually confined to wheelchairs) sings and claps hands along with her. We have found varying degrees of enthusiasm for this activity depending both on the mental and physical health of the patient. Those patients who are not too severely disabled by time or by illness seem to reflect the pleasure of the group leader. More and more nursing homes are coming around to the realization that geriatric patients need more than just bed-and-board. Arm exercise is the cheapest and best way to keep patients alert and healthy. It costs practically nothing. It requires no added space. Highly skilled (and costly) personnel are not necessary to teach or lead arm exercises.

Such exercises, however, must never be considered a sport suitable only to the older person. The infant who holds on to the top rail of the crib while he struggles to walk around is an early practioner of the art. The youngster who climbs a tree, casts a fishing rod, or plays Little League baseball is a slightly older pupil in the school of good health. The tennis player and the shooter of basketballs have grown even wiser and more experienced.

At any time in life, from early youth to advanced old age, arm exercises contribute to health, pleasure and longevity.

CHAPTER VIII

Now See How Much Better You Feel

There is no question that people who use their arms vigorously enjoy greater longevity than those who allow disuse atrophy to set in at an early age. One does not need the example of a Toscanini, a Stokowski, a Chagall or a Michelangelo to prove this point. One can cite the many cases of ordinary Vermont farmers, Turkestan peasants, or the host of tailors and pressers whose life span has extended for ninety or more vigorous years.

Although medical science has emphasized leg jogging for more than a decade, this emphasis is misplaced and warrants immediate correction. After much study and evaluation, there is still no firm evidence that jogging increases your life span. Furthermore, compared to arm jogging, running is immensely more dangerous. Each day the list of instances where running has caused disability and even death grows longer.

For example, a thirty-one-year-old runner recently showed up at the University of Colorado Medical Center with his face flushed, itching and swollen. He also had giant welts or hives all over his body. A study of this patient showed that hives broke out each time he ate shellfish prior to running. The patient was allergic to shellfish but his allergy did not usually bother him and caused no rash or disability. It was brought out only by strenuous running and it was both annoying and incapacitating.[1] Although it is usually unwise to make a generalization from a particular instance, runners would be well advised to avoid shellfish (or whatever else they may be allergic to) before attempting a strenuous workout.

Sudden and unexpected deaths have been reported in runners and joggers and some doctors postulate that these deaths have been due in most cases to ventricular fibrillation (a fast, irregular heartbeat) in which the heart quickly "electrocutes" itself. Yet doctors are still at a loss to determine which joggers are *likely* candidates for sudden deaths and so can be forewarned to avoid running. Preliminary stress-testing on stationary bicycles has proved *nothing!*

At the First Department of Medicine the University of Helsinki, for example, a team of doctors recently pretested a group of men, including active joggers, sedentary persons and those who had suffered heart attacks. The results proved baffling. After all their tests, the doctors could only report the following:

"Thus, our present state of knowledge leaves us in a most unhappy situation, where ventricular premature beats of similar outlook might be both an indication and a contraindication for prescribing physical exercise, because differentiation between non-life threatening and life-threatening ventricular premature beats *has not been satisfactorily clarified.*"[2] (My italics.)

Summarizing a recent report in the *New England Journal of Medicine, Newsweek* magazine headlined its article: Stress tests: lots of false alarms. A group of medical experts under the direction of Dr. Thomas J. Ryan at University Hospital in Boston tested 1,464 men and 580 women "to determine how well the stress test detected disease." A good correlation was found when the doctor suspected coronary artery disease. In other words, the stress test simply confirmed what the doctors already suspected! On the other hand, the test issued false alarms for 12 percent of the healthy men and 54 percent of the healthy women. Specially to be noted is that these stress tests concerned leg exercise with practically no involvement of the arms and hands.[3]

There is no question that some health benefits result from physical activity. Recent statistics from the Framingham (Massachusetts) Heart Study, conducted over the past twenty-five years by the Boston University School of Medicine showed that the incidence of heart attacks decreased as physical activity increased. This was especially true for men, less valid for women. Exercise, however, was not the only factor in preventing heart attacks. Clearly, other things such as diet, life style, tobacco use, temperament and obesity all must be taken into consideration. Yet even when it comes to physical activities, which ones are good? Which are bad?

Running, of course, can be exceedingly hazardous, especially for *novice* runners. A recent report by Drs. Peter G. Hanson and Stephen W. Zimmerman of the University of Wisconsin Center For Health Sciences highlights the likelihood of exertional *heat stroke* in apparently normal but inexperienced runners.

The Wisconsin doctors state: "Organized road races are a growing source of episodic heat injury. Many of the popular annual distance events have recently attracted 2,000 to 8,000 participants. The highly motivated novice runners are particularly vulnerable to exertional hyperthermia in warm-weather road races."[4] In other words, beginners who attempt long-distance running in hot weather had better be most careful. If muscular strains and tears don't get them, heat stroke can.

Far more serious is the finding that marathon runners may have severe, even fatal, degrees of hardening of the coronary arteries. Mention has already been made of the autopsy findings in the case of Clarence Demar who had problems with his heart valves rather than with his coronary arteries. Yet in a 1979 report in the *New England Journal of Medicine,* four autopsied cases are cited in which *marathon* runners were found to have severe coronary artery disease. The ages of the victims, all men, ranged from twenty-seven to fourty-four. Doctors studying these cases concluded unhappily that "marathon running cannot ensure protection from coronary atherosclerosis or fatal coronary artery disease."[5]

The *New England Journal of Medicine* also contained the statement that "physicians who recommend ambitious exercise programs for their patients must remember that proof that his approach will prevent or even delay cardiovascular death is not yet available."[6] The best advice is that if you enjoy running (and have your doctor's approval), then run for enjoyment. It *may* or *may not* promote health.

There is no question, however, concerning the longevity of those who exercise their arms instead of their legs. We have already looked at the incredible records achieved by orchestra conductors like Toscanini, Von Karajan, Stokowski, Fiedler and Eugene Ormandy. Even younger conductors such as Leonard Bernstein, Seiji Ozawa, Naozumi Yamamoto, and Zubin Mehta display a vitality that is extra ordinary for their years. They are all practically ballet dancers on the podium before the orchestra. Although their arm motions are predominant, there is a comparable rhythm to the syncopated movements of their entire bodies.

If we turn from music to sports, it is apparent that the best athletes are the rowers. This is especially true if we define *best* as *conducive to greatest longevity.*

We have already mentioned Stan Mullins, the sixty-eight-year-old Harvard graduate who races his scull every day. Even more remarkable is Leverett Saltonstall, former senator from Massachusetts and captain of the Harvard crew that won the Great Challenge Cup at Henley in England.

In 1914, led by Captain Leverett Saltonstall, Harvard's junior varsity crew became the first American eight to win the Henley cup. It was an achievement that made all Americans proud. Greater still was the fact that *fifty years later,* in 1964, *every man* who pulled an oar in the victorious Harvard crew, including the coxswain, was still alive. They all returned to Henley for a nostalgic reunion at the Thames Regatta.

In no other athletic event, except rowing, has ever anyone been able to get a whole team together for a celebration of a victory that they have achieved *fifty years* earlier. The rowing exercise that this Harvard crew, for example, had engaged in half a century earlier had served them well the rest of their lives.

The main reason for the great therapeutic success of *arm* exercising is the fact that there is a close and intimate relationship between the circulation of the arms and the circulation of the brain.

The heart pumps its blood out through a larger artery (the *aorta*) that comes out of the top part of the heart, towards the arms and head. Just as the aorta turns to the left (in most individuals) as it heads downward to the trunk and legs, it takes a U-turn, forming a well-circumscribed arch. As it starts its turn on the right, an arterial branch takes off (the *innominate* artery) which quickly divides into two arteries, the *subclavian* which goes to the right arm and the *carotid* which goes to the right side of the face and the right side of the brain.

As the arch of the aorta then turns downward on the left side, two branches lead off: the left *subclavian* that goes to the left arm and the left *carotid* that goes to the left side of the brain and the left side of the face.

It is apparent, therefore, that any exercise that increases the circulation to the arms must, because of these anatomical relationships, increase the circulation to the brain. Anatomists have long believed that the remarkable evolution of man's brain was related to the prehensile thumb and the subsequent use of tools. Hand action was believed to be the stimulus for increased neuron formation in the brain. It is equally likely that arm and hand exercise and the resulting increased *circulation* was the stimulus to increased brain growth and intelligence.

Now we are not claiming that everyone who jogs with his arms is going to become a genius, but there is no question that such exercise leads to a sense of well-being that the jogger may not experience. In many parts of China, for example, Tai Chi exercises are practiced every morning with almost religious intensity. Arms, legs and other muscles are used in synchronized activity for stimulating the *whole* body. Millions of devotees of this form of Oriental exercise can attest to the therapeutic value that it brings.

It is about time, then, that we molded our lives and the lives of our children along the examples that have proved successful. The overweight, muscle-bound football player hardly ever enjoys a long, effective life. Better examples are violinists, pianists, orchestra conductors, swimmers and rowers. In other words those who use their arms the most live the longest!

It is never too late to start exercising your arms. Whether you are a youngster just starting school or a senior citizen, the time to get started is now.

Just practice a few minutes each day. Start with the easy exercises and work up to the more difficult ones. You will certainly feel better and probably live longer.

Let's go. To arms! To jarms!

---

[1] R.N. Maulitz; D.S. Pratt; and A.L. Shockett, "Exercise-Induced Awaphylatic Reaction to Shellfish," *Journal of Allergy and Clinical Immunology 63* (1979): 433-34.

[2] M.T. Viitasalo; R. Kala; Antti Eisalo; and P.I. Halonen, "Ventricular Arrthythmias During Exercise Testing, Jogging and Sedentary Life," *Chest,* July 1979, pp. 21-26.

[3] "Stress Tests: Lots of False Alarms," *Newsweek,* August 13, 1979, p. 40.

[4] Peter G. Hanson and Stephen W. Zimmerman, "Exertional Heat Stroke in Novice Runners," *Journal of the American Medical Association,* July 13, 1979, p. 154.

[5] T.D. Noakes; L.H. Opie; A.G. Rose; and P.T. Kleynhans, "Autopsy-proved Cornary Atherosclerosis in Marathon Runners," *New England Journal of Medicine,* 301:2 (July 12, 1979): 86-89.

[6] D. Rennie, and N.K. Hollenberg, "Cardiomythology and Marathons," *New England Journal of Medicine,* 301:2 (July 12, 1979): 103-104.

Bibliography

Wayne A. Leadbetter, M.D. "Getting Ahead Of The Injury" Clinical instructor in Orthopedic Surgery George Washington University, Emergency Medicine, Page 27, June 15, 1979.

William L. Haskell, PhD. "How Does Your Body Run?" Clinical Assistant Professor of Medicine Stanford University School of Medicine Palo Alto, California Emergency Medicine page 43 June 15, 1979.

Roy H. Maffly, M.D. "Running Out Of Water" Professor of Medicine Stanford University School of Medicine Palo Alto, California Emergency Medicine page 57 June 15, 1979.

Page 47: "Autopsy-Proved Coronary Atherosclerosis in Marathon Runners" by T.D. Noakes, M.D., L.H. Opie, M.D., A.G. Rose M. Med, P.T. Kleynhams, N. Med New England Journal of Medicine 301:2 86-89 (July 12, 1979).

Page 48: "Cardiomythology and Marathons" D. Rennie, M.D. and N.K. Hollenberg, M.D., Ph.D. New England Journal of Medicine July 12, 1979 Page 104 (Vol. 301 No. 2).

Index